Nutritional Strategies to Correct PCOS and Infertility

By

Lynne D M Noble

Independently published December 2024

About the Author

Lynne Noble was born in 1953 in Huddersfield, West Yorkshire. From a very early age, Lynne showed an interest in nutrition and genetics avidly reading any books that she could get her hands on at the time.

Initially, Lynne studied orthopaedics but events led her to work with the elderly mentally infirm. Here, her interest in neurodegenerative disorders and pain syndromes developed.

Lynne undertook rigorous programmes of study, completing her Cert Ed., (FE) BSc (Hons) and Adv. Dip Education simultaneously before moving onto her M.Ed.

From there she took further demanding programmes in Human Nutrition, Pharmacology, Neuroscience, Genetics and Immunology. During this time, she was given many prestigious awards for her academic work. It was noted then that Lynne was not afraid of tackling difficult subjects.

She began her law degree but ill health prevented her from pursuing this. However, in this time, she moved from being a foster parent to adoptive parent.

She has been instrumental in setting up projects in the community for disadvantaged groups.

She is a member of the Guild of Health Writers.

Now retired, she lives with her husband in a historic Georgian riverside town in the West Midlands. She enjoys gardening, watching her husband bowling and researching.

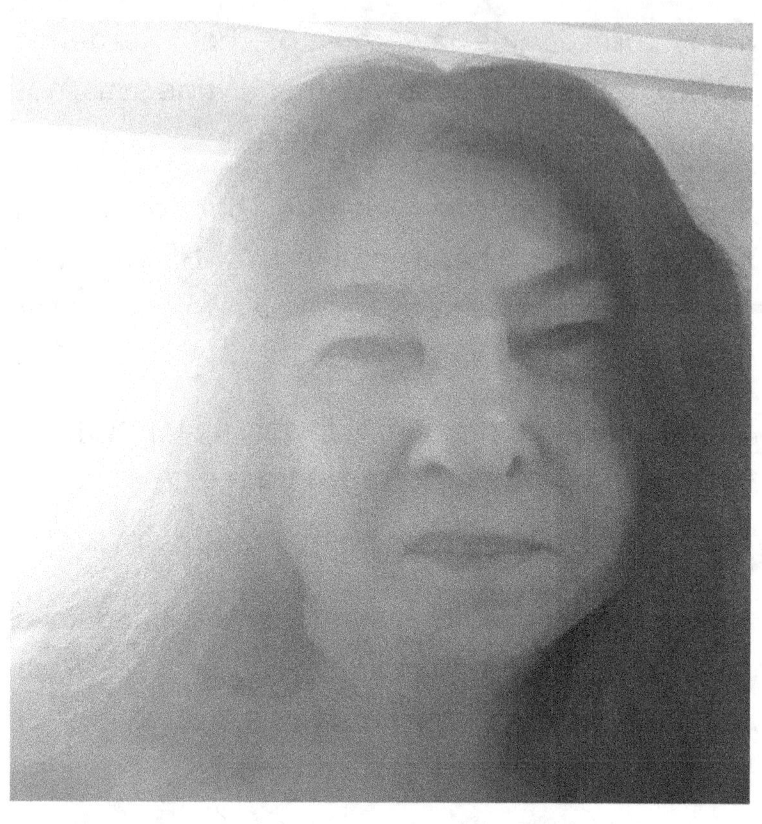

Author Lynne Noble at home

https://quintessentiallylynne.weebly.com/nutritional-medicine.html

Table of Contents

Preface

A Diet to Correct PCOS and Infertility came about because I had so many people contact me asking me to help in this respect. Polycystic ovarian syndrome, to give this condition, its full title, has even affected my family and so I have more than a mild interest in it especially as I can see those who have not yet been diagnosed with it, experiencing the same symptoms as those who had been.

More recently, my husband had been shown a picture of an ancestor; a masculine looking female with square jaw be whiskered and obese who had remained, to her distress, childless.

Then I recalled Audrey who lived in Almondbury where I lived my early married life. Like my husband's relative, she was large, with square jaw which was liberally supplied with thick wiry hair. She was gentle and kind but rarely went out as she felt a freak. She was alone and spent Christmases alone. Just prior to the last Christmas that we saw her she mentioned that she would not suffer another Christmas alone.

She kept her word; she committed suicide on Christmas Eve, alone.

PCOS has many distressing insults attached to it one of these being that those with PCOS find it difficult to become pregnant. Many remain childless but from that transition of hope to the realisation that pregnancy may never happen, what should be a joyous and spontaneous intimate act becomes something that is regulated and is monitored by the medical profession. Now, there are three or more in the marriage; privacy no longer exists and close relatives anxiously ask questions about what is, after all, something that is sacred between partners.

Many relationships unfortunately falter because the intensity of attempting to conceive, takes away from the beautiful relationship that used to exist before it became such a task. It seems impossible to give energy to both; trying to conceive when it no longer a spontaneous act is soul destroying.

Many of my clients have described the lack of sympathy, from the medical profession, for their childlessness. 'Go home and lose weight,' they are informed knowing full well that losing weight with PCOS does not happen however much you try. That is another insult that this condition delivers; the weight gain which deposits itself around your abdomen so that nothing looks right on you. That extra effort you made for a whole week shows a loss of zero pounds no matter which way you stand on the scales.   Your friend, who offered to be your dieting partner to encourage you, lost a whole 4lb on the same diet, for the same time period. It doesn't seem fair; it isn't fair especially when so little help is offered.

Then there are the menstrual irregularities which can include:

Heavy periods

Intermittent bleeding

Absent periods

Extended periods

And as ovulation is irregular or absent then infertility is an issue.

PCOS is also linked with oily skin and cystic acne, thinning hair, male pattern baldness and hair growth following the male pattern which is excessive.

Sleep apnea is common with PCOS. Sleep apnea results in people stopping breathing for some seconds. Sufferers who suffer frequent pauses find that they are brain fogged the following day, often falling asleep if they should sit down for a moment. Depression is common.

The skin also darkens. It becomes thicker, with velvety patches appearing under the arms or breast and in the groin. Some may appear on the back of the neck, too. What causes this? Is it related to insulin resistance? If we could address the insulin resistance could this address the POCS. There is much to explore and much to answer but hopefully at the end of this book, there is more knowledge and more hope using nutritional medicine, so let us begin.

What is Polycystic Ovarian Syndrome?

PCOS is not just condition; it can be divided into one of 4 different types. Each type has its own underlying cause which requires different treatment from the others.

Sometimes there is overlap and it is possible to have more than one type.

10% of women will suffer from PCOS in one form or another.

The most common one is the insulin resistant PCOS but there is also:

Post pill and post pregnancy PCOS

Inflammatory PCOS

Adrenal PCOS

As the insulin resistance type of PCOS affects approximately 70% it seems right to start with looking at this one first.

Insulin resistance is also known as hyperinsulinemia where insulin levels are higher than normal. This occurs when cells are not as responsive to insulin and the body attempts to address this by increasing the amount produced.

Hyperinsulinemia is linked to abdominal fat, an inability to lose weight, sugar cravings and brain fog.

High insulin levels increase androgen. Androgens are sex hormones which help develop and maintain male characteristics such as facial hair.

In women, androgens help with the development of pubic hair as well as axillary hair.

Androgens are produced in the ovaries, testes and adrenal glands. Testosterone is one such androgen.

When there is an excess, not only are insulin levels higher but:

High blood pressure

Dyslipidaemia

Vascular irregularities

also occur

Fasting blood sugar levels are normally undertaken by the family GP to see whether insulin resistance is present. Normal levels are under 60 pmol/l.

It is highly likely that there will be a familial tendency to type 2 diabetes as well as cases of metabolic syndrome, high blood pressure other family members with PCOS. Lipoedema may also be found.

Whenever we are dealing with insulin resistant PCOS the response to insulin must be improved and this can be achieved in a number of ways.

Reducing sugar intake is desirable although this can be difficult given the sugar cravings that those with insulin sensitive PCOS have. It is important to have enough thiamine (vitamin B1) in the diet because this helps turn glucose into energy.

Thiamine cannot do this without enough magnesium to activate it and it does need the help of all the B complex in achieving this.

Therefore, the protocol for insulin resistant PCOS at this point is:

100mg thiamine

300mg of magnesium (citrate or glycinate are better ones for this purpose)

A good vitamin B complex

Thiamine helps modulate mood and aids sleep. It also – along with the B complex - helps prevent furring of the arteries and thus is one mechanism able to lower blood pressure.

Low carbohydrate diets are an aim but do not necessarily work. The body seems to give in for a while so that a little weight loss may occur, but it seems to jump back for no reason at all.

Two other supplements which are recommended for this type of PCOS are N-acetylcysteine and inositol.

N-acetylcysteine (NAC) is a metabolite of the non-essential amino acid L-cysteine. It is widely used in those with lung problems such as pulmonary fibrosis and COPD. It is also used to good effect when there has been an overdose of paracetamol taken for which it is the antidote if caught in time.

NAC is also a powerful antioxidant where research shows it can help improve:

Insulin resistance

Reduce inflammatory process

Balance hormone levels

Increase fertility

Improve liver function

Metformin is a prescription medicine often prescribed for PCOS. It helps to improve insulin resistance but it has negative gastro intestinal side effects. Further, it inhibits thiamine which is an important nutrient in tackling PCOS.

Thiamine deficiency is rife, greatly affects the quality of life but is little recognised.

Various studies have shown little difference between the administration of metformin and NAC on improvements in PCOS symptoms.

Increase in fertility

For those who have been desperately trying for a family, NAC offers some hope. For example, a review carried out in 2015 in the Journal of Obstetrics and Gynaecology investigated whether the 910 participants had significantly improved fertility; it was found to be so with ovulation showing significant improvement and better pregnancy and live birth outcomes.

Like Metformin, NAC is also able to improve menstrual regularity.

Part of the positive impact of NAC may well be due to its ability to restore hormone balance.

A later 2019 study found that those women who took 1800mg/day of NAC compared to the Metformin group (1500mg daily) for a period of 24 weeks showed greater reduction in their testosterone levels.

The antioxidant capacity of NAC helps reduce the damaging effects of inflammation which has been found to be higher in those with PCOS.

Non-alcoholic fatty liver disease is associated with PCOS, high triglyceride levels and insulin resistance but NAC is effective in lowering the risks from this condition.

As already stated, NAC is a metabolite, an end product of L-cysteine so you won't find it in food as such but increasing foods containing L-cysteine will help. All animal proteins contain this amino acid and vegetables in the onions family such as red and brown onions, leek and garlic all contain reasonable amounts.

NAC can be bought as a manufactured supplement and, in matters of PCOS, it may be beneficial to supplement with it as it is unlikely that you will be able to reach the doses recommended for PCOS. Be guided by the recommendations on the packaging - which tend to be generous – as well as the amounts used in the study comparing the benefits of NAC at 1800mg daily for improvements in fertility.

Inositol is another nutrient that has potential benefits for those with PCOS. Also known as myo inositol it helps improve the cellular response to insulin and thus is effective in increasing insulin sensitivity. Therefore, the pancreas does not need to secrete as much insulin.

Inositol, via a reduction in insulin levels, helps lower the level of androgens and this will help reduce the appearance of acne and unwanted hair known as hirsutism. This occurs alongside increased ovulation rates.

Other studies have found that myo-inositol reduces the cardiovascular risk associated with PCOS.

In a similar way to NAC, it can also restore the regularity to the menstrual cycle.

4000 mg per day of myo-inositol in two divided doses is recommended for PCOS although doses of up to 15000mg have been given without negative impact.

One of the side effects of taking myo-inositol may be weight loss which may be due to its effect in lowering insulin sensitivity. However, it is useful to reduce fat in the diet of the pro-inflammatory seed oils as these change the microbiota in the gut.

Studies on rats found that those fed on high fat diets became obese and showed insulin resistance. However, the type of fat was not mentioned.

 Prior to seed oils becoming popular, people did not show the apple shaped abdominal obesity; people on diets using saturated fat from animals had the typical pear shaped figure which was deemed to be healthy.

Indeed, the popular Atkins diet demonstrated that high fat diets did not put on weight nor does animal fat change the gut bacteria to one that is unhealthy.

With PCOS, it is far healthier to swap the poly unsaturated fatty acids – omega 6 – which are highly inflammatory in nature for the saturated animal fats like:

Butter

Dripping

Lard

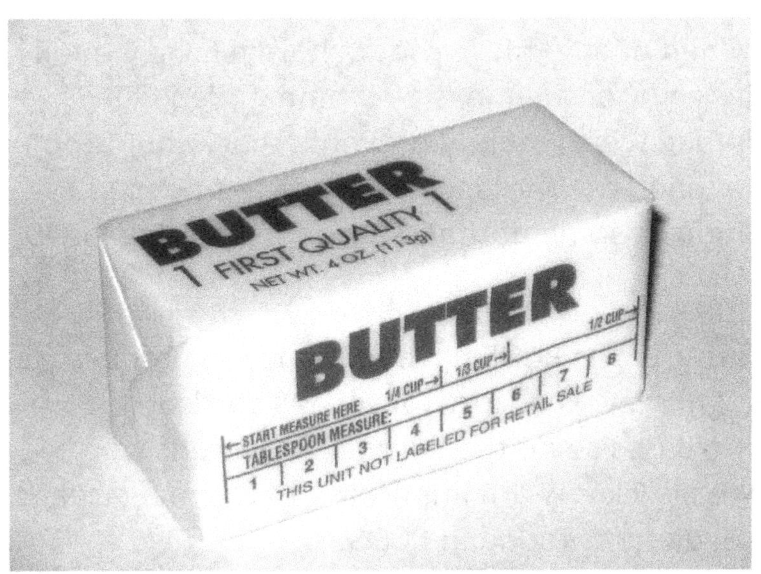

Butter is a far healthier fat to use when you have PCOS than the inflammatory seed oils.

Vitamin C and PCOS

Before you think that such a common vitamin, oft associated with alleviating infections, can possibly help with PCOS, then you need to realise two things

Vitamin C is a powerful antioxidant which is required in an inflammatory condition like PCOS.

When people think about vitamin C they think in terms of the measly recommended daily intake which merely prevents scurvy but is not taken in the therapeutic quantities needed to address some of the issues underpinning PCOS.

Sufferers of PCOS have tendency to produce higher levels of cortisol and, as cortisol increases so do the adrenal androgens which we now know are implicated in the menstrual regularities found in PCOS.

Vitamin C is regulatory in this respect helping the adrenal glands modulate the amount released and thus normalise testosterone levels.

Vitamin C is a single chain antioxidant and is able to help maintain normal progesterone levels.

Progesterone is needed for proper fertility and normal menstrual cycles.

A little known fact is that just prior to ovulation, extra vitamin C is needed as it is post ovulation. Without this process, it is doubtful whether pregnancy could occur or be maintained as normal ovulation would not occur.

Ascorbic acid also stimulates oxytocin known as the 'cuddle hormone' for its ability to engender feelings of trust and bonding.

Generous levels of vitamin C present in the ovaries may be responsible for collagen synthesis: This is required for follicle and corpus luteum growth, egg ripening, as well as repair of the ovary post-ovulation and pregnancy support. Problems with collagen formation, ovulation and ovarian repair due to vitamin C deficiency may contribute to the development of ovarian cysts.

A dose of 750 to 1000mg of vitamin C has been shown in studies to raise progesterone in women. There is a unique benefit of progesterone for women with PCOS as it can block the enzyme 5-alph-reductase, which is involved in the metabolism of testosterone. Additionally, progesterone is the hormone that helps to regulate the monthly cycle, facilitate ovulation, and reduce PMS and menstrual cramps.

Magnesium

Magnesium is a vital mineral which also has a role to play in those with PCOS who are magnesium deficient.

It has numerous roles to play in the body alongside addressing insulin resistance so any, or all of these conditions may also occur alongside it.

Involved with proper nerve and muscle function including the alleviation of spasm.

It is used in the synthesis of bone helping to retain its density and prevent osteoporosis.

It helps to maintain a normal blood pressure

It activates vitamin D and thiamine, two essential vitamins required for nutritional therapy for PCOS

Magnesium is an essential component in the synthesis of DNA and RNA.

How does magnesium work to prevent insulin resistance?

Magnesium is required to regulate electric activity and insulin secretion in the beta cells which are located in the pancreas. As magnesium deficiency is common then attention must be paid to diet to ascertain that it contains good amounts of magnesium containing foods (see below)

However, although the majority of studies show that magnesium supplementation can improve insulin sensitivity in type 2 diabetes, PCOS and obesity, one study did not. Nevertheless, not all patients with PCOS have to be magnesium deficient as this is not the only factor which is implicated in insulin sensitivity.

Diuretics will certainly strip your body of magnesium as will medications like antibiotics and proton pump inhibitors.

Magnesium is found in a wide range of foods including:

Green leafy vegetables

Whole grains

nuts

it comes in supplement form of which there are many varieties including:

magnesium citrate

magnesium glycinate

magnesium taurine

magnesium carbonate

magnesium sulphate.

Magnesium citrate is the most popular one bought as it is easily absorbed and not as highly priced as some of the others.

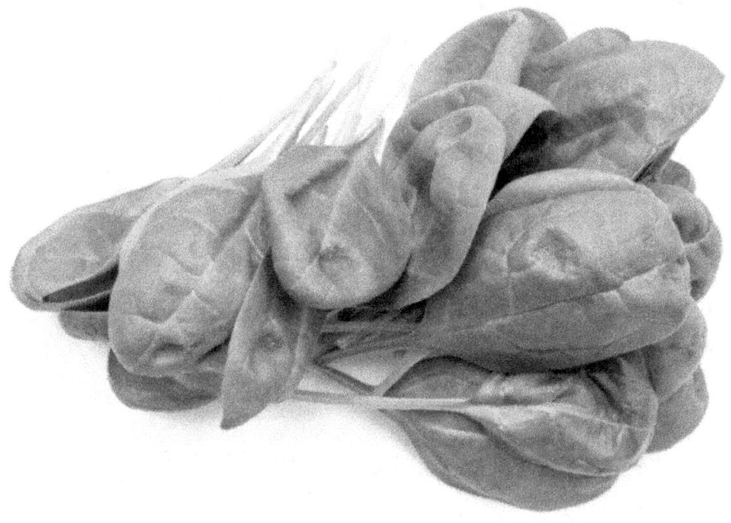

Spinach: a good food to help raise magnesium levels

Chromium

Like magnesium, chromium is an essential mineral which directs how insulin helps the body to regulate blood sugar levels.

If the body cannot make enough insulin or cannot use it due to insulin resistance, then an excess of sugar remains in the bloodstream. This can cause all sorts of problems such as:

Furring of arteries (atherosclerosis)

Poor wound healing

Obesity

Chromium deficiency is very common especially in the:

Elderly

Those whose diets are high in simple sugars

Pregnant women

Those involved in excessive exercise

Alongside elevated blood sugar levels there is an increase in triglycerides. Triglycerides are the commonest type of fat found circulating in the blood stream and are used as a form of energy. If this energy is not needed then they are laid down as fat in the body and can be a risk for diabetes, PCOS and heart disease.

Although the main source of chromium is wholegrains, it can also be found in:

Lean meat

Brewer's yeast

Cheese

And some spices like black pepper

Again, some research supports chromium as being useful in insulin resistance and others do not; nevertheless, it cannot be repeated often enough that many other deficiencies can contribute to insulin resistance, not just chromium.

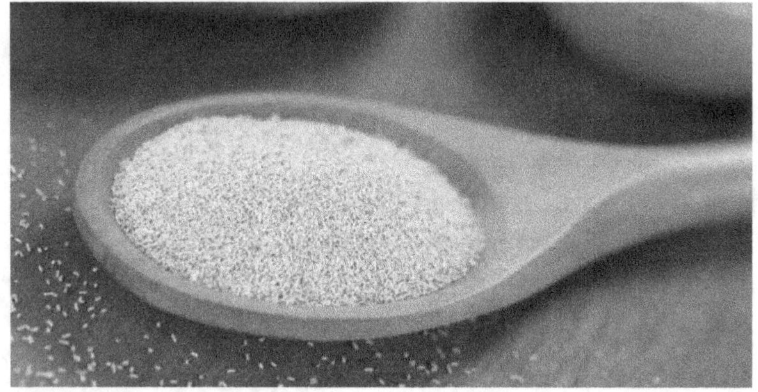

. Brewer's yeast contains chromium

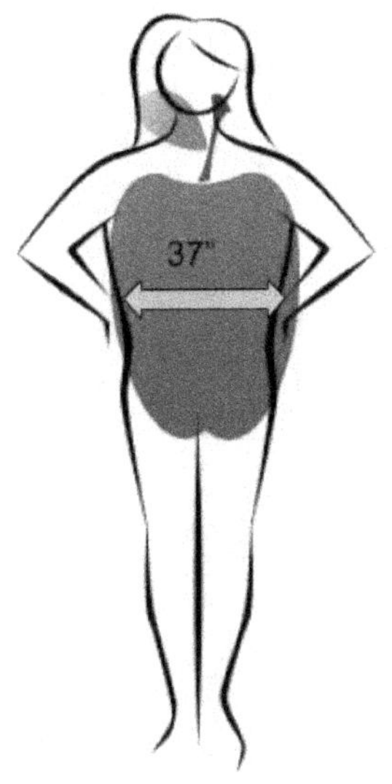

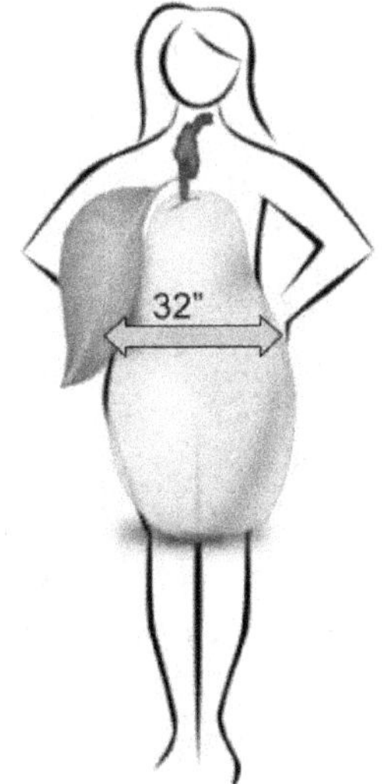

Apple

**Upper-body obesity
(android-apple shape)**

Pear

**Lower-body obesity
(gynoid-pear shape)**

Apple shaped obesity occurs when there is insulin resistance so it frequently seen in those with PCOS

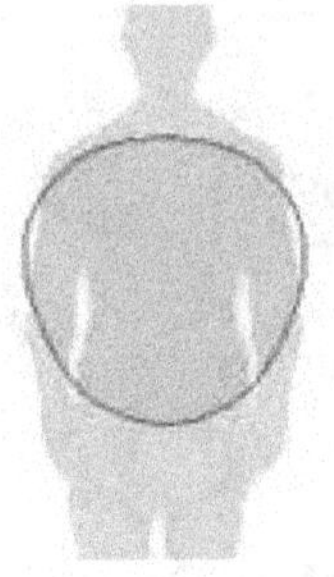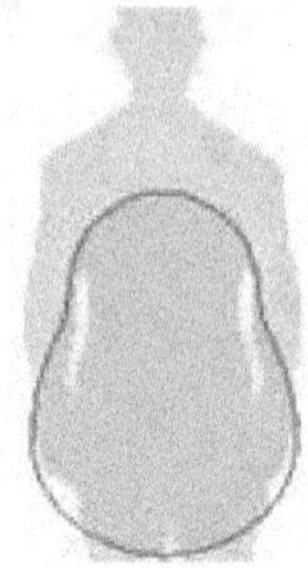

Abdominal fat deposits press on organs and is one contributor to constipation which is one of the common side effects of PCOS.

Berberine is one of the newer treatments for PCOS. It is a yellow substance found in plants such as goldenseal and Oregon of grape. These plants have been used in Chinese and Ayurvedic medicine for a long time.

These plants have a wide range of application including:

Skin diseases

Infections

Digestive problems

Currently, it has said to have efficacy with weight loss and its usefulness for diabetes is also being studied.

With weight loss, the evidence is not conclusive although there have been some significant results in those taking 1g of berberine daily for 8 weeks.

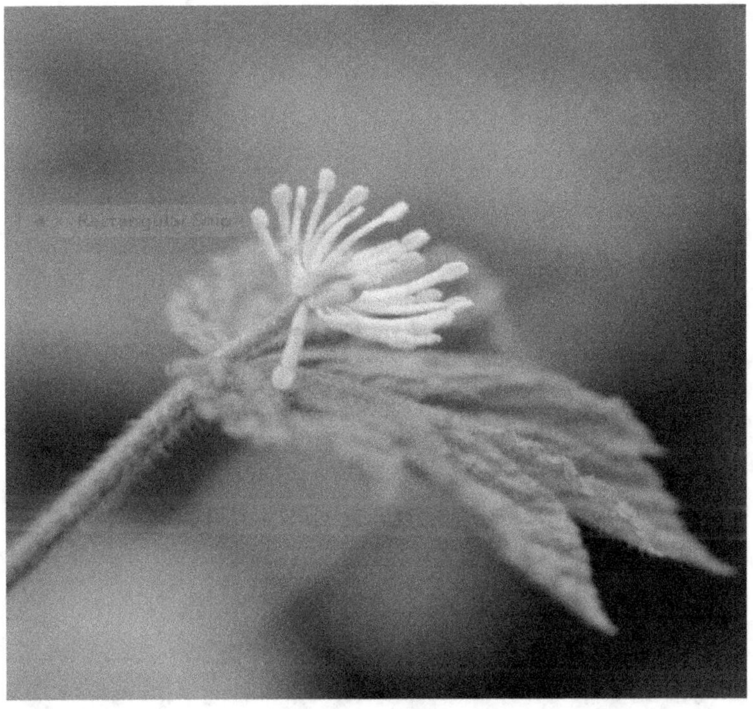

Goldenseal; a plant which may help with the treatment of PCOS

Studies have shown reductions in BMI and weight but not all studies are consistent. However, given genetic diversity, this should not be surprising.

As berberine has been used mainly in Asia then this is where the majority of studies have taken place on those whose ethnicity may well be very different from those reading this book.

There are some studies that show that babies exposed to berberine may build up bilirubin in their brains so using berberine, when breastfeeding, may be unwise.

Berberine has a number of impressive actions when combatting insulin resistance including:

Reducing inflammatory chemicals including C-reactive protein which is used to measure acute inflammatory responses. Interleukin 6 is another chemical messenger which is implicated in inflammatory responses but is inhibited by berberine. Indeed, berberine is said to be as effective as Metformin, the diabetic drug in addressing insulin resistance.

Berberine is also said to aid an increase in insulin production as well as decreasing cell resistance to insulin.

Receptors, of course, are needed to grab onto insulin; when berberine is take the expression of insulin receptors is increased.

Berberine also improves beta cells activity. Beta cells secrete insulin.

Finally, berberine is able to regulate lipids in the blood by inhibiting the synthesis of a proteolipid protein. Proteolipids are just proteins which are attached by covalent bonds to lipids.

Choline is a fairly new kid on the block when it comes to nutrients. It has a fairly impressive history in that those babies, whose mothers had higher levels of choline in their diets when pregnant, tend to have superior cognitive functioning.

Some say that choline is categorised as a B vitamin and others say that it doesn't quite fit that description; what we do know is that it is need for fertility and a healthy pregnancy. Low levels are associated with non-alcoholic fatty liver disease of which a significant proportion of those with PCOS suffer from.

Choline is able to donate a methyl group which has the ability to affect gene expression. It is also vital in the synthesis of hormones and the special group of chemicals found in the brain known as neurotransmitters.

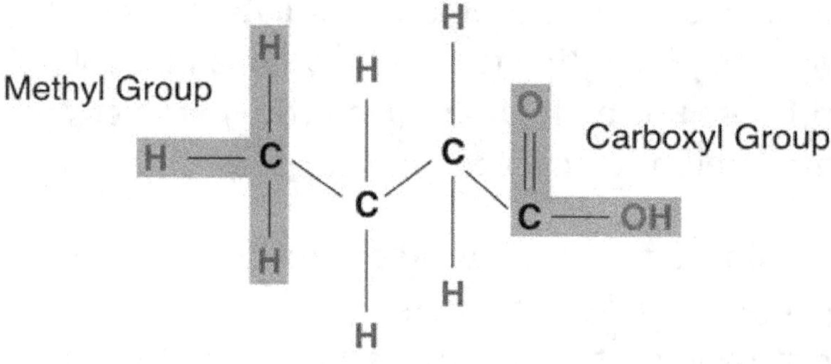

Choline's ability to reduce the risk of heart disease, is not disputed although it requires good amounts of folate to achieve this and metabolise the amino acid homocysteine which is harmful and only required for a short time in the methionine cycle.

In a study[1] of 150 women with PCOS, three groups either took;

Metformin with clomiphene citrate or

Choline and inositol and clomiphene citrate or clomiphene citrate.

It was found that the Metformin group were more likely to have regular cycling.

However, in the Metformin group and the inositol/choline group there was no difference in the rates of conception which were higher than those in the clomiphene citrate group alone.

---

[1] The Egyptian Journal of Hospital Medicine (April 2023) Vol. 91, Page 4802-4807

Choline is found in:

Chicken liver

Salmon

Dairy

eggs

Grass fed steak

Chicken and turkey breast

Whole grains/nuts/seeds

Cruciferous vegetables like cauliflower

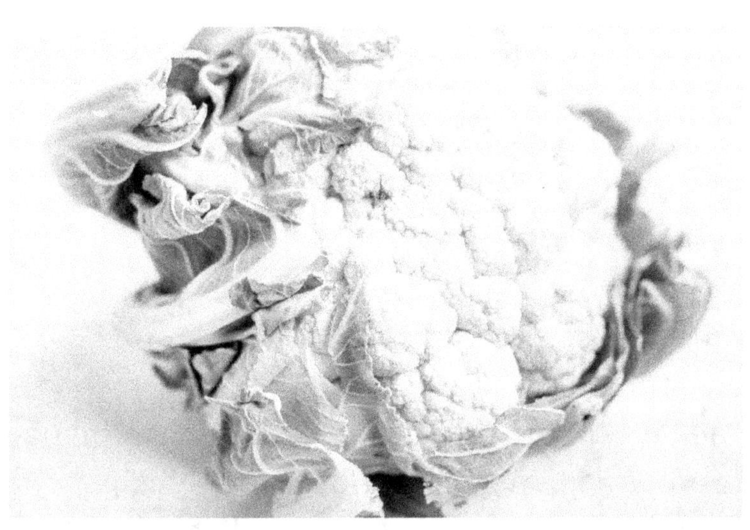

Cauliflower is a source of choline

The recommended daily intake of choline is as follows:
Adult female: 425mg
Pregnancy: 460mg
Breastfeeding 550mg
It is reported that only about 10% of pregnant women have sufficient intake of choline in the US.

Choline, like folate (synthetic form = folic acid) helps to prevent neural tube defects.

Choline is also able to reduce the risk of pre-eclampsia.

Adiponectin and vitamin D

The fat cells produce an inflammatory hormone know as adiponectin. Not only does it help regulate appetite and satiety but it increases insulin sensitivity, regulates metabolism and blood pressure.
There is a link between lower vitamin D levels and low adiponectin levels. In this respect, lower vitamin D levels are a risk factor for insulin resistance.

Sufferers of PCOS have generally been found to have lower levels of vitamin D which is significantly correlated with insulin resistance.

Vitamin D deficiency is likely to be the number one nutrient deficiency for many reasons.

It is a fat soluble vitamin but the advent of no fat and low fat diets have increased the potential risk of vitamin D deficiency.

People with PCOS tend to be overweight and many will opt for a reduced fat diet.

The main non-food source of vitamin D is through the action of the sunlight on the skin. For this we need sunlight, which has been a rare sight at the time of writing and further, we do need cholesterol for this process. It goes without saying that those on cholesterol reducing medication are at a significant disadvantage for making vitamin D.

Those prescribed statins tend to be the older end of the population who will not make vitamin D as effectively because age makes us slightly less efficient at doing this than when younger.

The sun, a miracle vitamin D producing body

Increasing vitamin D levels also decreases the levels of fasting plasma glucose (lowers the risk of diabetes) and thus decreases testosterone levels.

In a study of women with PCOS who had less than 20 ng/ml of vitamin D - evidencing a vitamin D deficiency - some were selected, at random to receive 50,000 IU's for 8 weeks given as a single dose weekly.

It was found that those who had been given the supplement had decreased their fasting plasma glucose levels which lowered their risk for becoming insulin resistant.

It was also found that sufficient vitamin D levels raised adiponectin levels which helps reduce the tendency to obesity as well as other risk factors such as heart disease.

The standard recommended daily dose for those with PCOS is 400IU's and is woefully inadequate for this condition. The level of 400 IU's was originally arrived at as the minimum amount required to prevent rickets which was rife in the 1950's; the minimum amount required to prevent PCOS, in those with a genetic propensity to it, is much higher.

Vegetarians and those whose diet is heavily plant based will have to supplement vitamin D if they do not see the sun much; this would apply to office workers, for example. The only plant based source of vitamin D is to be found in irradiated mushrooms, that is, mushrooms that have been left in the sun to absorb its rays.

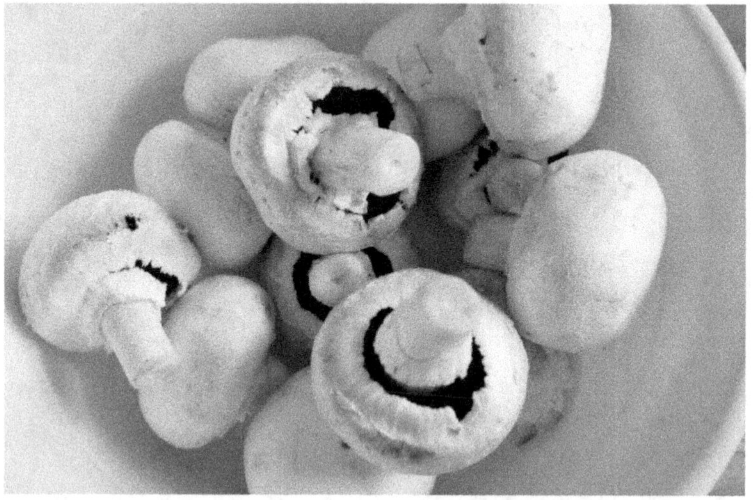

Irradiated mushrooms are a reasonable source of the inactive form of vitamin D. that is vitamin D2

The form of vitamin D found in mushrooms is D2, an inactive form which requires to undergo a number of stages in the body before it is activated. It also requires magnesium in order to be able to achieve this. Magnesium deficiency is also very common; given its hundreds of roles in the body, it is important to rectify this deficiency as soon as possible.

Food items which contain vitamin D3 are limited but include:

Oily fish: salmon, sardines, mackerel
Animal fats like lard, dripping and butter
Limited amounts in cheese
Egg yolks

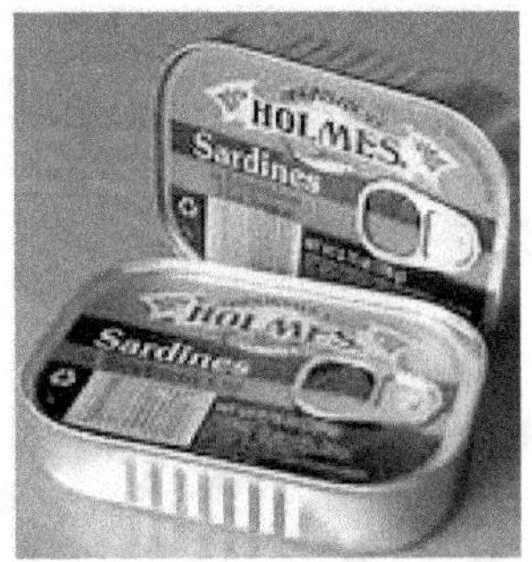

Tinned sardines; a source of vitamin D3

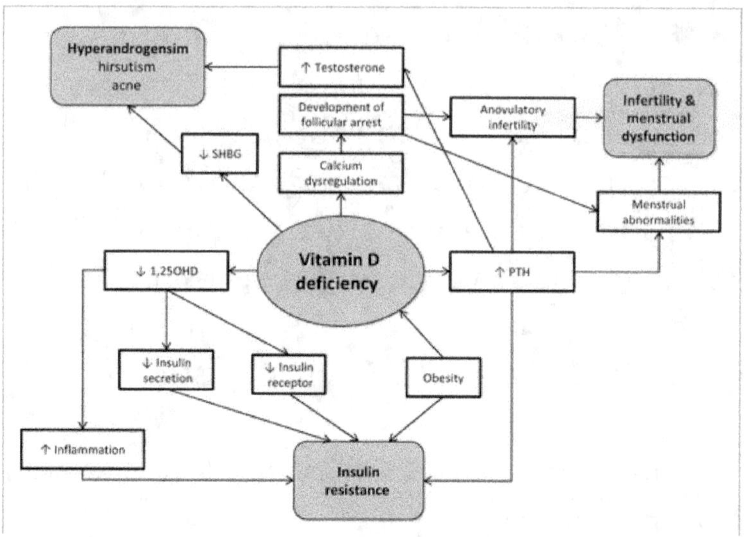

The role of vitamin d in the pathogenesis of PCOS[2]

Vitamin D and hirsutism

The greater the vitamin D deficiency, the more likely that the individual with PCOS would have hirsutism.

---

[2] https://onlinelibrary.wiley.com/doi/10.1111/j.1365-2265.2012.04434.x

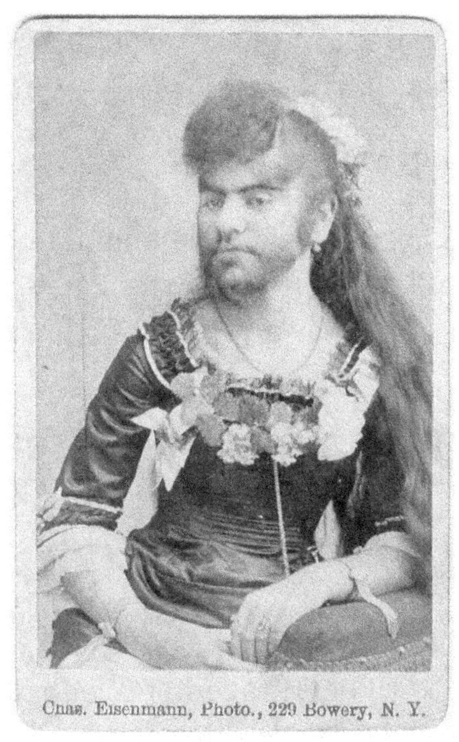

The bearded lady: androgen dependent hirsutism

Reference ranges for vitamin D

- <25 nmol/L – DEFICIENT.
- 25-50 nmol/L – INSUFFICIENT.
- 50-75 nmol/L – ADEQUATE.
- >75 nmol/L – OPTIMUM.

The management of PCOS through adequate levels of selenium

Studies of the impact of selenium insufficiency are limited. Nevertheless, selenium does affect metabolic profiles of those with PCOS.

In a 2014 study entitled:

Metabolic response to selenium supplementation in women with PCOS: a randomised, double-bind, placebo-controlled trial

By Mehri Jamilian, et al

70 women with PCOS, aged between 18-40 years old were given 200ug selenium supplements daily for weeks.

At the start of the study, fasting blood samples were taken and again at the end of the study to ascertain, glucose, insulin and lipid levels.

It was found that:

Serum triglycerides decrease significantly

Insulin resistance markers improved

Very low density cholesterol markers improved. The amount of selenium in food very much depends on the soil it is grown in as many soils are selenium depleted.

Selenium is vital for reproductive capacity and just one brazil nut provides more than the recommended daily intake of selenium.

Selenium also prevents damage to tissues.

Nevertheless, selenium is toxic if taken in too high a dose. The symptoms of selenium toxicity are:

Muscle tremors

 dizziness

loss of hair

stomach upset

The sources of selenium, apart from brazil nuts are:

Animal protein including shellfish and liver

Whole grains such as brewer's yeast, nutritional yeast flakes

Mushrooms

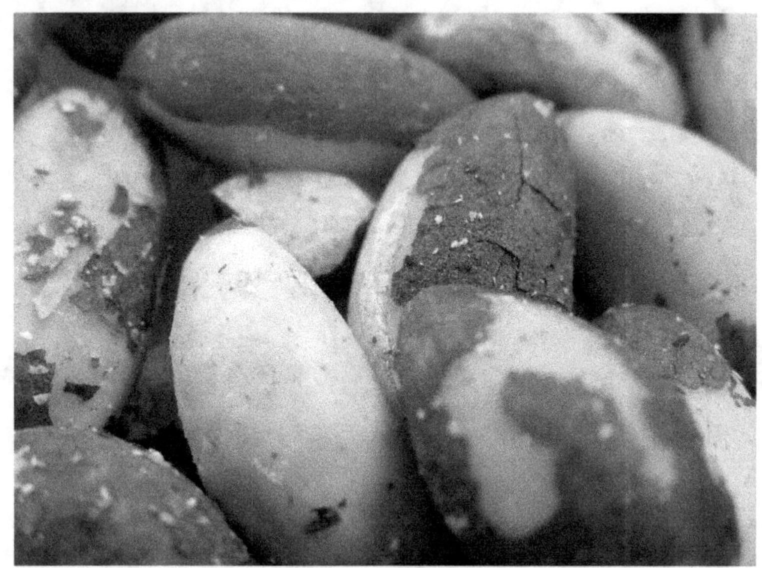

Brazil nuts: a good source of selenium

Histamine intolerance, oestrogen dominance and PCOS, the connection

One of the main causes of histamine intolerance are hormonal imbalances. The hormonal imbalance that we are mostly interested in here is the one known as 'oestrogen' dominance which simply means that the levels of oestrogen and progesterone are not in harmony with each other

Oestrogen dominance is the main culprit in PCOS development. Sufferers of PCOS are more likely to have had premenstrual syndrome and are more at risk from breast cancer and uterine fibroids.

The insufficiency of progesterone becomes a problem as it is intimately connected with the function of an enzyme known as diamine oxidase (DAO).

Without DAO you cannot break down histamine in the body and the excess oestrogen is aids the release of histamine from mast cell in both the uterus and ovaries.

More outward manifestations of excessive histamine are:

Skin issues like hives

Hay fever

asthma

The gut issues, bloating, chronic fatigue, insomnia and headaches are all PCOS symptoms which could be attributed to excess histamine.

Oestrogen levels are higher during the first part of the cycle so the potential for symptoms of histamine intolerance are more likely to occur then or at least with greater severity.

Although antihistamines are normally taken for histamine intolerance, antihistamines have unwanted side effects like:

Excessive and rapid weight gain

Somnolence

Brain fog and inability to learn

Constipation and

an increased risk of Alzheimer's disease.

Increased risk of infection

They work by blocking the histamine receptors on each cell. However, an alternative to antihistamines, which do not have the above side effects, is vitamin C in therapeutic doses i.e. in the region of 1g (1000mg daily). It works slightly differently than antihistamines and regulates the amount of histamine produced whilst its other benefits include:

Collagen synthesis

Normalising bowel movement

Better mental health through the synthesis of serotonin, the 'feel good' chemical

Better immune function

Possible weight loss as it helps use fat for energy; this also increases body temperature so that you are less likely to feel cold in winter.

While vitamin C significantly increases oestrogen in post-menopausal women who are on hormone replacement therapy, in those who are premenopausal, it helps to increase progesterone levels.

Vitamin C is really good for balancing hormones and alleviating PCOS and this includes whatever type of PCOS is manifested.

Therapeutic doses are generally higher than we can hope to get from our daily food intake. We must treat high dose vitamin C as a (nutritional) medicine.

In order to increase the enzyme DAO, which would in turn lower histamine by breaking it down, we could increase the intake of olive oil which is one of the best external sources of this enzyme. Thus, in matters of histamine we can:

Table showing how to reduce histamine levels

antihistamines	Blocks histamine receptors (not recommended due to the side effects
Vitamin C in therapeutic doses	This reduces the amount of histamine and is recommended
increasing DAO	Useful as it helps to break down histamine, although too much may result in increased gut motility; in matters of PCOS where constipation is a general symptom, this may be used therapeutically
Lowering foods containing histamine. See list at the end of this book.	Useful although it may be difficult to balance the diet especially if you do not like being in the kitchen

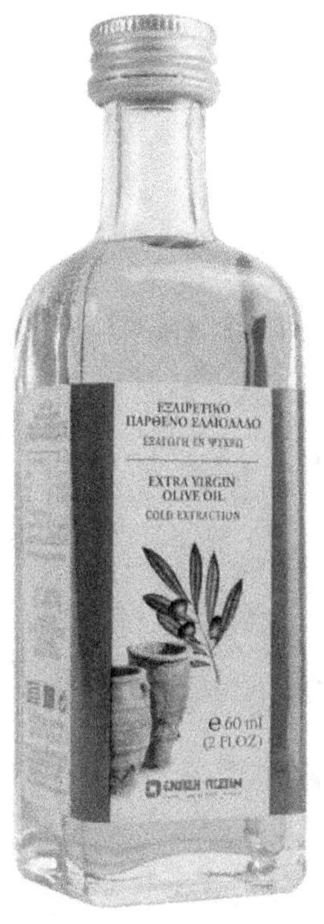

Contains DAO which helps to break down histamine

Finally, although this book is about the dietary aspects underpinning PCOS, it is necessary to remind people that regular exercise is important to help improve insulin sensitivity. Exercise is needed to help burn sugar as well as build muscle. In matters of PCOS, we should use all the tools we have to combat its effects.

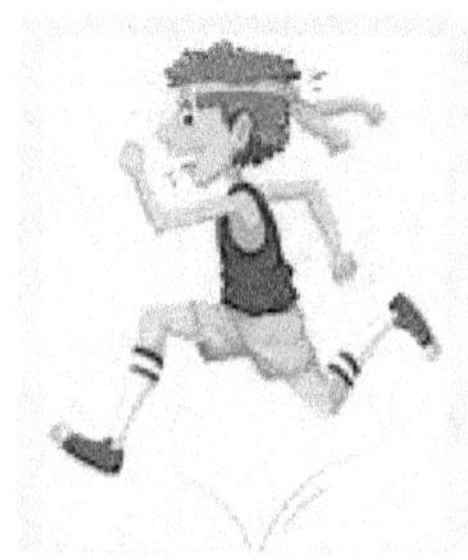

PCOS after taking birth control pills

Unfortunately, when people are prescribed the birth control pill, they are not generally informed that it is a risk factor for PCOS which becomes evident once the pill is stopped.

Sadly, one of the main reasons for stopping the pill is to start trying for a baby. The advent of PCOS makes this event difficult to achieve.

The symptoms of PCOS were not evident prior to taking the pill but acne, irregular periods and weight gain are evident soon after.

It appears that pills involving synthetic progestins are the culprit. Once released from the inhibitory effect of the contraceptive pill, it appears that androgens go into full swing although insulin resistance is not a symptom.

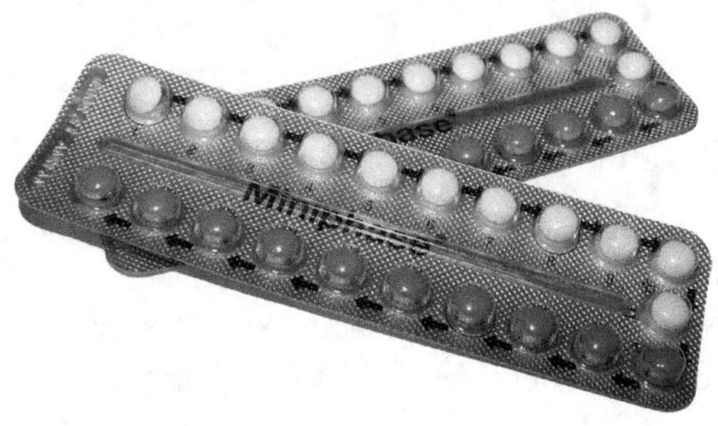

Some contraceptive pills can cause temporary PCOS

This type of PCOS will settle down eventually.

Reducing stress is important especially as many will be planning a pregnancy.

Vitamin C, the B complex and L-theanine will help manage the post contraceptive pill time.

L-theanine is an amino acid which is useful for controlling stress and anxiety but without the sedating effects that other inhibitory amino acids have.

Small amounts of found in tea which is why tea appears so refreshing. However, L-theanine can be bought online and at some health food shops as a powder or granular form. Amino acids are useful as they are absorbed in the stomach and into the bloodstream as soon as they reach the stomach, that is, in a matter of seconds.

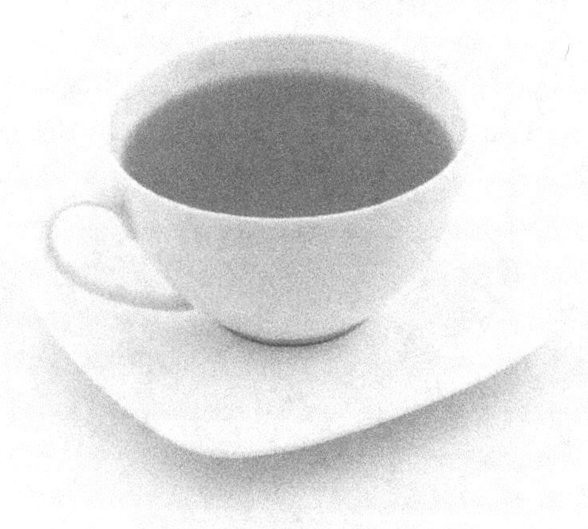

Tea contains theanine which helps reduce stress.

Adrenal PCOS; a sign of our times?

As the pace of life speeds up and people have little time to adapt to the changes, the potential for a prolonged stress response and adrenal PCOS, increases.

In the adrenal response, it is the androgen DHEA-S that tends to be implicated.

The full title of DHEA-S is dehydroepiandrosterone-sulphate. It is a steroid hormone which is produced in the adrenal glands. It is converted into androgens and oestrogen.

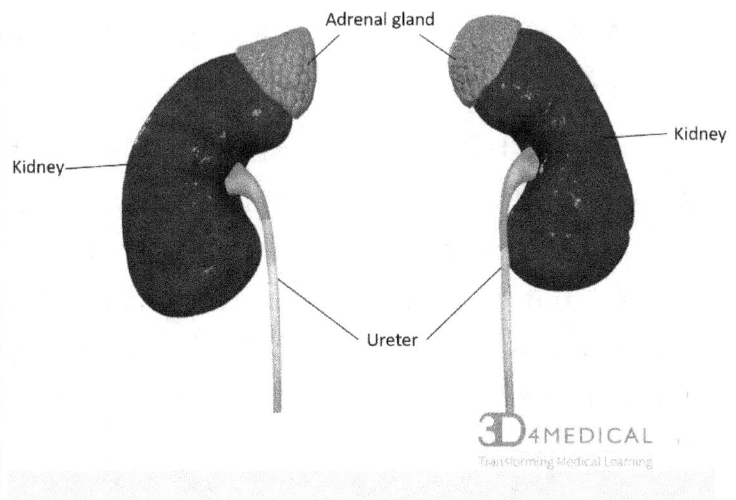

This type of PCOS is often missed because the two hormones which are – and indicate PCOS - testosterone and androstenedione   are not elevated in this case. It is normally DHEA-s but this is not routinely tested for. Pantothenic acid is required in the synthesis and metabolism of steroid hormones (of which vitamin D is a well-known one.

At times of stress, it is prudent to increase foods containing pantothenic acid as the adrenal glands will require it in huge amounts.

Pantothenic acid is also needed for the production of energy from fats, proteins and carbohydrates. Without this energy, cells simply cannot function properly.

Fortunately, the 'pan' at the beginning of the pantothenic suggests that it is found everywhere and that many foods contain it. It is unlikely that an insufficiency of pantothenic acid is high on the list of nutritional deficiencies but it is more likely that those with adrenal fatigue are.

Excellent food sources of pantothenic acid are:

Organ meats: liver and kidney

Meat in general: beef, pork, chicken, lamb turkey

Dairy

Vegetables in general

Like most nutrients pantothenic acid needs to be activated in order to carry out its function properly and this requires the nutrients:

Vitamin A

Vitamin B6 - pyridoxine

Vitamin B12

Vitamin B9 – folate (synthetic form is folic acid but not everyone can utilise folic acid)

Vitamin B3 - niacin

Once activated pantothenic acid becomes panthenol

Vitamin A is fat soluble and found in full fat milk

Egg yolks

The fatty part of meats

Lard

Dripping

Butter

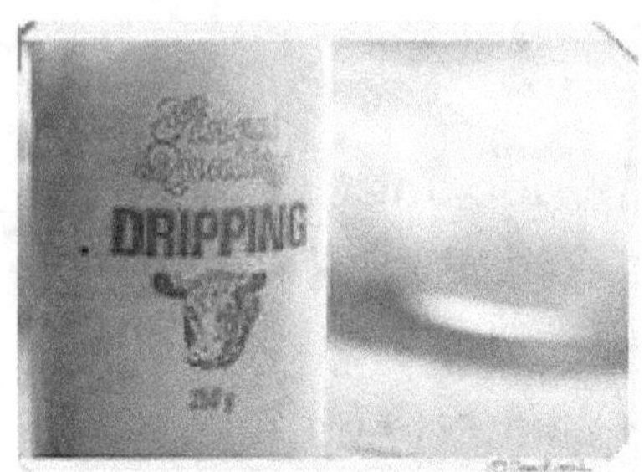

Dripping is full of the fat soluble vitamin A which is required to activate pantothenic acid

Vitamin A as a lipid soluble vitamin is involved in steroid synthesis and has antioxidant activity too. Vitamin A is well known to prevent PCOS from occurring in the first place but the very low fat diets do not allow for adequate absorption of vitamin A.

It is likely that the low fat diets are preferred by those with PCOS because they are likely to have a higher Body Mass Index with greater abdominal mass in the first place. This is counter-productive. Eating fat does not necessarily lead to weight gain as the popular Atkins Diet will evidence.

Even if the type of PCOS is not the common insulin resistant type there will still be some degree of insulin resistance involved.

Looking at the principles of the diet for insulin resistance would be useful; this would include regular exercise.

Both vitamin A and D have steroid function and it may be helpful to understand a little more of what this means.

Britannica defines steroid hormone as

any of a group of hormones that belong to the class of chemical compounds known as steroids;

they are secreted by three 'steroid glands' the

adrenal cortex

testes

ovaries and

during pregnancy by the placenta

All steroid hormones are derived from cholesterol. They are transported through the

Basically, hormones are chemical messengers being synthesised in limited tissue and then travelling to where they are needed.

As well as acting as a steroid, vitamin A, acts in nutrient capacity. Thus it is both steroid and vitamin.

It is vital for metabolic activities and for proper growth and development. Children will no doubt recall being told to eat their carrots up as it was good for night time vision. This was often followed up by the joke that you never saw a rabbit wearing glasses.

As it is possible to obtain the precursor of vitamin A form carotenoid (vegetables which are often red or orange in colour) then there are both animal and plant sources. However, in order for the plant source to be absorbed well, it is better taken with a little fat. Hence the practise of adding butter to vegetables; it wasn't just for the taste but to enhance absorption.

In addition to producing sexual steroids, it is also required for:

Spermatogenesis

Conception

Formation of the placenta

Cell division

All of which have some bearing on a successful outcome for a pregnancy.

A deficiency of vitamin A does lead to a decrease in the testicles and ovaries.[3]

This is just the tip of the iceberg when we look at what vitamin A is capable of benefitting.

Jang et al 2017 suggested that,' *PCOS, one of the most prevalent ovarian endocrinopathies in reproductive aged women globally, may,*

---

[3] O'Byrne & Blaner, 2013

Is it that conception does not happen easily for those with PCOS but that pregnancy does happen but nutritional deficiencies abort this before pregnancy tests are even considered?

In Rapid Response; missing link[4] this paper looked at PCOS, the pill and mineral deficiencies. It was found that common nutritional deficiencies were:

Zinc

Magnesium

Manganese

Chromium

Copper

B complex and

Essential fatty acids

---

[4] https://www.bmj.com/rapid-response/2011/10/30/polycystic-ovarian-syndrome-pill-and-mineral-deficiencies

The authors remarked that 'essential nutrient status is largely ignored by medical professionals.

There is a link between zinc and magnesium deficiency and ovarian cysts. The use of ovarian and pituitary stimulating drugs makes these worse. Further, there is a link between these two deficiencies and aversion to food as found in anorexia nervosa and binging. However, nutrient deficiencies have far wider impact on PCOS and fertility than this study's remit.

Some research by Clagett-Dame and Knutson, 2011 found that it was possible to avoid foetal atrophy by taking rats with vitamin A deficiency and injecting them with retinol. This had to occur before the tenth day of pregnancy.

It may be useful to look at further functions of the retinoids. These include:

Embryogenesis,

Immunity

Cell division

 Proliferation

Oocyte maturation

Retinoid signalling also influences meiosis which takes place in the foetal ovarian germ cells.

The authors of the study concluded that:

'the relative vitamin A levels in females during conception and pregnancy are an important factor in determining the success of reproduction and a vitamin A shortage may result in absolute infertility prior to implantation, fetal resorption, or deformity.' [5]

---

[5] Clagett-Dame & Knutson, 2011

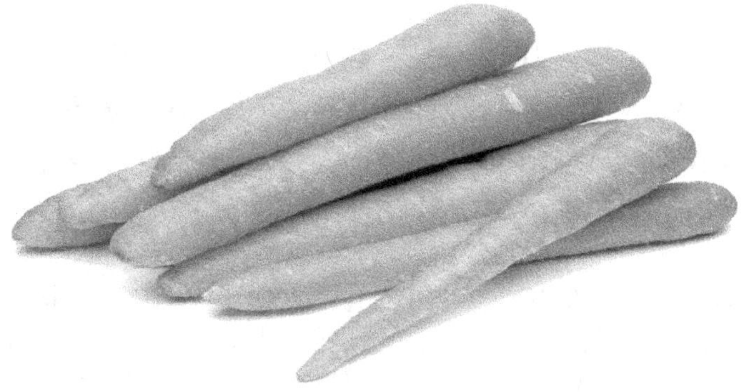

Carrots contain a precursor to vitamin A and could be an aid to address infertility

It has also been found that prescribing vitamin A to women with PCOS also aids insulin sensitivity and improves hyper insulinaemia.

Maybe, just maybe, PCOS is just a manifestation of a vitamin A deficiency and maybe it might be useful to see if there is a link between vitamin A deficiency and obesity.

As it is, there is; Zulet et al has reported that there is an inverse relationship between obesity and vitamin A intake in healthy adults.

This study also found an inverse correlation between similar findings in those who were morbidly obese. This form of obesity – also known as class III obesity is defined as a body mass index that is 40 or above. Another way of classifying morbid obesity is by stating it is over 100 pounds above your ideal weight.

There are a couple of things wrong with using BMI. Firstly, the BMI was not originally invented as a way of classifying weight. Secondly, the ethnicity of an individual also confounds any use that the BMI might have.

By all means, apply it loosely but it is not gospel.

In those who are obese there are certain markers such as:

Interleukin 6 is elevated

Leptin is elevated

serum amyloid A is elevated

Tumour necrosis factor is elevated

Although the above are more likely to accurately reflect obesity, the cost involved of undertaking such tests are more than simply calculating the BMI.

In matters of determining the cause of PCOS, women may be short changed and denied the chance of motherhood on cost alone.

The vitamin A metabolic pathway impacts on the regulation of insulin sensitivity. Yet when we are considering vitamin A as a potential cause of PCOS and infertility in general we are reminded that those preparing for conception or in the stages of pregnancy are informed that they must not eat liver as it is too high in vitamin A and may cause abnormalities in the developing foetus.

The form of vitamin A that is alleged to be the problem is the preformed vitamin A which is derived from animal sources. The recommendation is not to eat more than 25000mcg daily.

Testing for vitamin A deficiency involves measuring the amount found in blood. Levels between 20 and60 mcg per decilitre written as mcg/dl are acceptable. A severe deficiency is anything below this. However, this is a severe deficiency; even a mild deficiency could affect fertility and the manifestation of PCOS.

Inflammatory PCOS

We now come to our final type of PCOS, that of the inflammatory form.

There are two types of inflammation, acute inflammation which occurs at the beginning of infection and injury and is necessary to begin the process of healing.

This form should last no longer than 12 weeks, if it does then it is considered chronic inflammation which is pathological.

It is chronic inflammation that is found in this form of PCOS; this inflammatory process in the ovaries causes the ovaries to synthesise excessive testosterone.

Inflammatory forms of PCOS are indicated by some symptoms which aren't found in the other forms; for example, there may be 'itis' conditions like arthritis and joint pains, headaches and irritable bowel syndrome.

What there won't be will be signs of insulin resistance although caution here, there is no reason why more than one form of PCOS cannot co-exist and this can delay a proper diagnosis and appropriate measures and treatment to rectify.

There are simple blood tests which can be undertaken such as the C- Reactive Protein which can test for inflammation although this is used more for acute inflammation.

The erythrocyte rate (ESR) measures how rapidly red blood cells fall in a sample of blood and the rate at which it settles evidences whether inflammation is present or not.

Plasma viscosity looks at the viscosity of the blood; this increases during inflammation.

One inflammatory condition can be comorbid with many others so while it is not easy to see chronic inflammation affecting the ovaries, the presence of other inflammatory conditions may alert you especially if a planned pregnancy hasn't happened.

Metabolic acidosis is associated with PCOS and it is useful to understand what happens here and how it impacts other conditions.

A strategic response to the state of acidosis in order to reduce pain and inflammation

Acidosis is implicated in many disease states yet very few people have heard of it or how it may impact health. However, the systemic acid-base balance may be responsible for significant changes in the immune response. Imbalances may help promote and prolong immune dysfunction. Acidic states may support certain infections increasing their severity and length.

There are different forms of acidosis – metabolic and respiratory - which may impact the immune system differently.

 Metabolic acidosis can be further subdivided into types:

- lactic

- hyperchloraemic

Metabolic acidosis develops when too much acid is produced in the body or if the kidneys and lungs are unable to remove enough acid from the body. The pH of the blood should be around 7.4 and anything lower is referred to as acidosis whilst anything higher is referred to as alkalosis.

Lactic acid build up – which is one of the subgroups of metabolic acidosis – occurs after prolonged exercise. It is responsible for the 'stitch' pain that we feel after intense exercise.

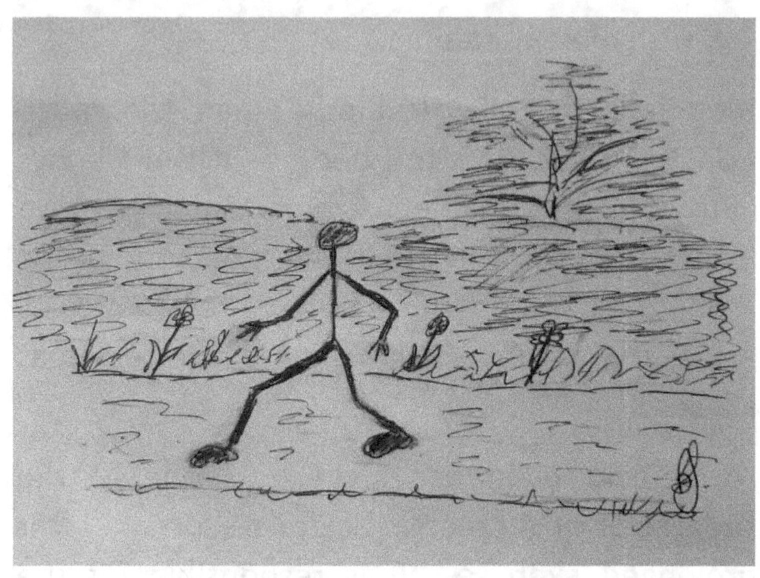

Intense or prolonged walking may result in lactic acid build up and metabolic acidosis

Hyperchloraemic acidosis occurs if when there is a decrease in bicarbonate concentration and an increase in chloride so that there is an imbalance of these two substances.

The bicarbonate can be lost for two main reasons:

- It may be lost from the gastrointestinal tract. One possible reason is that this may be due to the use of laxatives.
- a defect in the body which causes poor regeneration. For example, in chronic kidney disease the kidney loses its ability to synthesise ammonia, regenerate bicarbonate and excrete hydrogen ions.

Dietary causes of metabolic acidosis occur when there is an excess of fat or protein in the diet which is not balanced by bases such as calcium, potassium and magnesium. The acidic residues of protein produce subclinical or low grade metabolic acidosis.

Such a state may cause:

- kidney stone formation
- reduced bone mineral density and increased bone resorption
- loss of muscle mass
- chronic diseases such as type 2 diabetes, hypertension and non-alcoholic fatty liver

disease (all these three are associated with PCOS).

High blood sugar levels indicate that there is some form of insulin resistance or that the production of insulin is not adequate to allow glucose to enter the cells to be used as energy.

When insulin is inadequate then fats are broken down and form ketones which can be used as energy. This action can also produce a state of acidosis known as ketoacidosis.

Sodium chloride (salt) is reported to be an independent and causal factor for inducing metabolic syndrome. Salt is added in huge amounts to just about every tinned and packaged food item unless it has 'reduced salt' on the label. This will often then be sold at a grossly inflated price.

On many an occasion when I have investigated items masquerading as low salt, they are anything but.

We do need salt in our diet. It is vital for our health but there can also be too much of a good thing; as such it may cause imbalances in other electrolytes.

High salt diets are implicated in the progression of multiple sclerosis, for example.

The recommended daily dietary intake for salt, in adults, is one teaspoon per day. This equates to 2.4g of sodium.

In children it is age dependent:

1-3 years = 2g of salt daily (equivalent to 0.8g sodium)

4-6 years = 3g of salt daily (equivalent to 1.2g sodium)

Respiratory acidosis occurs when the lungs cannot remove enough carbon dioxide.

Excess carbon dioxide will cause the pH of the blood and body fluids to drop making them too acidic in the process.

Respiratory acidosis is caused by:

- Underlying disease such as asthma, COPD, sleep apnoea or pneumonia

- Conditions which can decrease the respiratory rate or inflation of the lungs. For example, obesity may prevent full expansion of the lungs.

Respiratory acidosis may cause symptoms such as:

- Anxiety
- Blurred vision
- Headache
- Agitation and restlessness
- Twitching
- Confusion

But this is not a definitive list.

As just about every chronic and/or painful condition will be underpinned by inflammatory processes, what can be done about it?

Researchers at the Medical College of Georgia discovered a nerve centre in a cell layer in the spleen that is responsible for the immune response and any inflammatory processes that occur throughout the body.

It is quelled by the addition of just 2g of bicarbonate of soda in half a glass of water taken for two weeks.

Bicarbonate of soda addresses metabolic acidosis and helps prevent the underlying and damaging inflammatory processes that accompany chronic conditions such as:

- Asthma
- Diabetes
- Obesity
- Arthritis

A report from the Netherlands in relation to asthma found that sodium bicarbonate (baking soda) reduced respiratory distress when given intravenously during a life threatening asthma flare up.

High blood acidity has a number unwanted effects in those with breathing disorders. It can:

- Reduce the effectiveness of beta agonist inhalers which are used to dilate the bronchioles.
- Cause the heart to contract more weakly

- cause rapid shallow breathing

The administration of sodium bicarbonate has been found to relieve bronchial spasm and allows the efficacy of bronchodilators once again.

Although there had been fears that the addition of sodium bicarbonate would raise blood carbon dioxide levels, this does not appear to be the case.

An analysis by Buysse and his team of 73 children with life threatening asthma found that the intravenous administration of sodium bicarbonate for those with acidosis resulted in a 'significant decrease in acidity' and further 16 patients experienced 'prompt improvements in respiratory disease and level of consciousness.

The anticipated increase of blood levels of carbon dioxide actually decreased significantly.

The researchers note that sodium bicarbonate was given to 14 patients in a last-ditch attempt to avoid putting them on a respirator, and only one of these subsequently required ventilation. All the patients survived.

Given these results, Buysse and her associates concluded that sodium bicarbonate was useful as an adjunctive treatment for life-threatening asthma.

Alongside asthma there are many comorbid conditions and these include:

- Rhinitis
- Sinusitis
- Gastro-oesophageal Reflux Disorder
- Obstructive sleep apnea
- Hormonal disorders
- diabetes

 which can all be helped by the administration of sodium bicarbonate.

Following on from the connection between asthma and diabetes, individuals with type 2 diabetes have similar risk factors to those found in:

- obesity
- endothelial dysfunction
- vascular inflammation
- dyslipidaemia
- cardiovascular complications
- end stage renal disease
- hypertension
- depression
- thyroid gland disease
- chronic obstructive pulmonary disorder

Sodium bicarbonate is cheap and easily obtainable from any supermarket and can be found in the baking department.

It is a superb medicine and deserves a place in every household.

Acidosis from any origin reduces leptin which plays a role in regulating body weight. Some asthmatics may find exercise and therefore weight control, difficult.

When bicarbonate (HCO_3^-) levels are low the kidneys upregulate an enzyme known as glutaminase.

This triggers cortisol production and raises blood pressure. It follows that a high protein, high fat diet or a diet that raises the blood sugar levels beyond its capacity to cope through insulin's regulating function, will inevitably raise blood pressure.

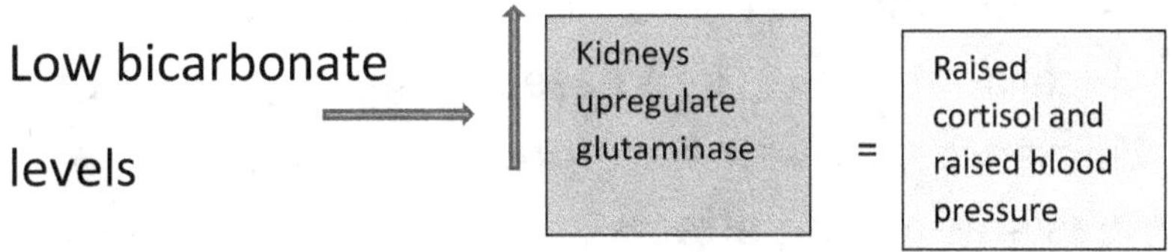

For those who like chemistry, it mediates this through the pituitary-adrenal cortex-renal glutaminase axis.

It has also been reported that upregulated cortisol bioactivity may be diet driven and promote insulin resistance in its wake.

Inflammation is implicated in asthma. It causes the lining of the airways to swell. It also helps produce mucus. Steroid inhalers may help with inflammation but as they increase blood sugar levels, they may also predispose to a pre-diabetic or diabetic state.

Extracellular acidosis helps the synthesis and release of inflammatory mediators especially tumour necrosis factor (TNF) and nitrous oxide (NO).

An alkaline diet – or the addition of sodium bicarbonate – decreases inflammation and increases growth hormone production. Thus it has anti-ageing effects.

The importance of optimum tissue pH can also be understood when you consider that the failure of local anaesthesia in inflamed tissue occurs when the tissue is in an acidic state.

Given that sodium bicarbonate can affect the severity, length and outcome of a disease, its worth should be more widely known. Indeed, in hospitals, it is often used intravenously to treat patients with severe conditions which have often worsened because they are in a state of metabolic acidosis which exacerbates the condition.

Pondering on this, this morning, I stated to my husband that we would be far better filling the salt pot up with sodium bicarbonate and sprinkling that on our meal.

Finally, and in relation to asthma and respiratory conditions, most respiratory bacteria and viruses thrive in acidic conditions. Thus by raising the pH of tissues, we can either prevent or reduce the impact of respiratory infection.

For long standing inflammatory conditions try:

Half a teaspoon of sodium bicarbonate in water twice a day for adults.

Continue for two weeks.

If the condition still hasn't cleared, reduce the daily intake to half of one teaspoon in water and sip throughout the day.

Continue this for one further week.

The inclusion of magnesium at 300mg daily would be helpful.

 Children from 5 years upwards should have half the adult dose.

For immediate conditions. For example, you feel a virus coming on, Arm and Hammer recommend:

6 X ½ teaspoonful taken in water at regular intervals throughout the first day.

4 X ½ teaspoonful taken in water at regular intervals throughout the second day

2 X ½ teaspoonful taken in water at regular intervals throughout the third day.

The Role of Fasting in Reducing Chronic Inflammation

A recent article that appeared in the Medical Express has highlighted the importance of fasting in reducing inflammation and chronic inflammatory disease.

As we have already discovered lymphoedema is a chronic inflammatory disease which has the potential to respond to such measures. Even more exciting is the discovery that fasting does not affect the immune systems response to acute infections.

Calorie restriction has long been known to improve inflammatory and auto immune disease but how this comes about has only been discovered.

Apparently, intermittent fasting reduces the release of monocytes. These are pro-inflammatory cells which are found circulating in the blood. During fasting these cells go into a dormant state and become less inflammatory in the process.

Monocytes are highly inflammatory and can cause serious tissue damage. Dr Merad[6] explained that increasing amounts of monocytes can be seen in the blood circulation of populations over the last few centuries due to different eating patterns.

Further studies have shown that people who have a poor diet can ameliorate the effects by the periodic use of a low calorie, plant based diet. This causes the cells to act like the body is fasting.

Longo[7] and colleagues conducted clinical trials where participants were allowed to consume between 750and 1l00 calories daily over a five day period. The diet contained specific proportions of proteins, fats and carbohydrates. The participants saw reduced risk factors for many life threatening diseases.

---

[6] https://medicalxpress.com/news/2019-08-fasting-inflammation-chronic-inflammatory-diseases.html

[7]

https://www.sciencedaily.com/releases/2019/03/190306171247.htm

'Fasting is hard to stick to and it can be dangerous. We know that the fasting-mimicking diet is safer and easier than water only fasting, but the big surprise from this study is that if you replace the fasting-mimicking diet, which includes pre-biotic ingredients, with water, we don't see the same benefits.

In mice studies, these findings were replicated. In the study one group of mice adhered to a four-day fasting-mimicking diet by consuming approximately 50 percent of their normal caloric intake on the first day and 10 per cent of their normal caloric intake from the second through fourth days. Another group fasted with a water based diet only for 48 hours. The fasting-mimicking diet was found to mitigate or reverse some of the inflammatory processes while the water based fast did not. This indicated that certain nutrients in the fasting-mimicking diet contributed to the positive changes found in the plant based fast.

The conclusion formed was that 'fasting primes the body for improvement, but it is the re-feeding that provides the opportunity to rebuild cells and tissues.'

PCOS is a condition which undoubtedly blights the lives of many, the importance of nutritional medicine in treating this condition cannot be underestimated.

Unfortunately, correcting a nutritional deficiency – or even investigating this potential avenue- does not take priority in mainstream medicine.

Prescriptions of strange sounding medications with side effects are given; patients with PCOS are told to 'go home and lose weight' as though this will solve the problems, as though it is all that simple. It isn't, not if the patient is being offered medication which does not treat the underlying cause.

Even if the patient is not trying to conceive, the metabolic disorder raises all sorts of risk for stroke, cardiovascular disease and should be treated on that alone.

The rotund shape which is typical of PCOS, the acne and hirsutism can be soul destroying and impact on mental. These symptoms themselves deserve compassion and a commitment to investigating the cause and a treatment plan.

Further useful information

List of anti-inflammatory foods

Turmeric

N-acetyl cysteine

Spices in general

Fresh fruit and vegetables

Omega 3 fatty acids found in oily fish such as mackerel sardines

Olive oil (due to the DAO content)

Green leafy vegetables have anti-inflammatory properties

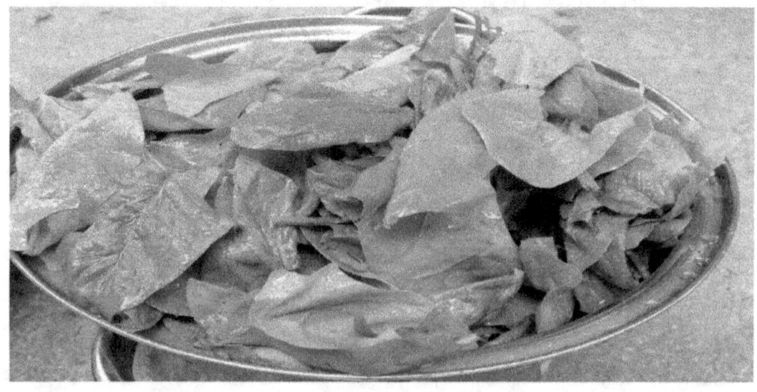

AVOID seed oils; they are inflammatory in nature and unfortunately added to just about every ready meal and processed food. Why this is, is anybody's guess. It simply is not needed. We have lived all our lives without this relatively new addition to our diets and our health has not improved because of it.

Avoid histamine containing foods such as:

Fermented foods

Alcohol

Canned, pickled and smoked foods like salami and bacon, smoked mackerel

Aged cheeses

Eggplant - aubergine

To reduce inflammation by keeping infection away.

Vitamin C is an excellent antioxidant but at very high doses it is effective as an antibiotic.

 Immune system cells called neutrophils, which are the first line of call when infection strikes, need to be activated; they are activated by sufficient vitamin C. Providing enough vitamin C for breakthrough infection helps reduce the likelihood of prolonged inflammatory processes throughout the body

Vitamin C levels drop rapidly when there is infection and to avoid this 'vulnerability period, research recommends 3g of vitamin C daily – in divided doses – for the first three days. If the infection does not appear to be waning then it is not detrimental to carry on at this level or even increase it as at 6g, vitamin C acts as an antibiotic.

Further 20,000 IU's of vitamin D plus 25mg of zinc and approximately 300mg, for three days, alongside the vitamin C generally stops infection in its tracks.

Conditions found alongside PCOS

Hashimoto's thyroiditis

Grave's Disease

Diabetes type 1 and type 2

Psoriasis

Systemic Lupus Erythematosus (SLE)

High blood pressure

High insulin levels

sleep apnoea

endometrial cancer

heart disease

non-alcoholic fatty liver disease

high cholesterol[i] but Cholesterol is a healing molecule and often levels which are deemed to be high is simply cholesterol responding to a need and does not, in any way, occur as a pathological warning which needs to be treated and reduced. Research shows that those people with what are deemed to be high levels of

cholesterol, are fitter, healthier, less likely to die
from a gastrointestinal or respiratory infection.
They also enjoy better cognitive function in
older age.

The amino acid profile in PCOS

The amino acid profile has been found to be significantly different in those with PCOS.

One such amino acid which has both antioxidant and anti-inflammatory action is histidine (don't confuse with histamine although it is a precursor to histamine.

Histidine is a precursor to another amino acid, glutamine which is found in significant amounts in the gastro intestinal tract.

A study which investigated L-histidine supplementation in women who had obesity and metabolic disorders assessed these markers:

Insulin resistance

Inflammation

Oxidative stress

Metabolic disorder

After 12 weeks of L-histidine supplementation it was found that:

There was lowered insulin resistance

Lower fat mass

Suppressed inflammation

Less oxidative stress

A rule of thumb for the recommended daily allowance of histidine is: 8-12mg per kilogram of body weight.

However, it has been found that in the US, Europe and Japan, the daily intake is nearer 30-35mg of histidine per kilogram of body weight.

It may be that those with PCOS are not following nutritionally sound diets.

Histidine is found in all animal proteins and most grains such as wheat, rice and corn.

Other books by this author include:

- The EDS and Hypermobility Syndrome Diet
- Alleviating Symptoms of EDS
- Gastroparesis
- The EDS recipe book
- The Lipoedema Diet
- The Lymphoedema Diet: reverse and repair lymphatic damage
- The Anti-Virus Diet
- The Asthma Diet
- The Reluctant Bowel
- The MND Diet
- Why we live longer with higher cholesterol levels
- A dietary connection for MACS, POTS and EDS
- Identity: a self-exploration workbook *
- Journey Through Pneumonia

- Parkinson's Disease: dietary changes that work
- The Thyroid Diet
- Shaken Baby Syndrome; an alternative explanation
- Beating back pain through diet
- The incontinence diet
- Allergy and intolerance; a dietary response
- Tap water and how to reduce its use
- https://www.amazon.co.uk/dp/B07TBHMV6N

*This book can be used alone or in small group work and is an excellent resource for those who are 'people helpers.'

Among many others

They are available on Amazon

Lynne has written a semi-autobiographical trilogy.

For the full range of books by this author, visit the author website on

https://www.amazon.co.uk/-/e/B07BPQZ5CD

https://www.amazon.com/-/e/B07BPQZ5CD

A percentage of the profits from the sale of these books go to support charities like the Exodus Project below.

The Exodus Project

My first introduction to the far reaching impact of The Exodus Project occurred when I was travelling around Cawthorne in one of their buses, visiting gardens.   A young lad was happily munching on a sandwich. He looked up briefly, pointed to the driver and said,' He's my second dad, he is,' then he returned to his sandwich without further comment

Such remarks are often very telling and so I arranged to meet Jackie Peel and Martin Sawdon, at the charity's premises in Barnsley. They set up the Exodus Project 20 years ago. They moved into their current premises – a redundant Methodist church - in 2010.

Both Jackie and Martin have been youth workers in their church. Martin worked in housing for the homeless in addition to working in learning disabilities services in institutional settings.

The work that the Exodus Project undertakes is of paramount importance to the communities it serves. These were former mining communities which became disadvantaged after pit-closures. Currently about 400 children attend mid-week activities from Monday to Thursday inclusive. These activities include dance, drama, craft, music, sports and games. In addition, there are weekend camps, cycle treks, outward bound activities, bowling and swimming. The children are taught valuable life skills including how to cook and bake. It is all about teaching children how to fulfil their potential and learn skills they will be able to pass onto the next generation.

The grounds, once overgrown, have been turned into a play- and camping - ground. A miniature railway is in the process of being installed.

Martin and Jackie have developed a unique model in that The Exodus Project goes beyond dispensing services. They are keen to build up relationships with the whole family and not just the child that attends the mid- week clubs. In addition, once children have reached the age of fourteen, they are invited to help out with the younger groups as junior volunteers. Once they reach the age of eighteen, they become adult volunteers. This model provides a constant supply of help from individuals who have benefitted already from attending such groups.

The   building is large and inviting. It is decorated with bold colours and has comfy seating. It is a real home from home; a haven for families who have been disadvantaged by the closure of the life force of its community.

Martin and Jackie have clear ideas about how they wish to develop the Exodus Project but the lottery funding which they benefitted from is no longer available. Sadly, they have had to close two of their clubs due to lack of funding. This decision wasn't taken lightly. They do have two charity shops which raises some money and they obtain some funding from outside organisations for the use of their facilities. However, this is clearly not enough to keep their clubs, weekend activities and building going to cater for the ever growing number of children who are benefitting from the work being undertaken here. Neither does it allow for future development.

Exodus do have a Just Giving page which can be found here if you wish to help further their work https://www.justgiving.com/exodus

In addition, you can keep up with activities on their Facebook page here

https://www.facebook.com/search/top/?q=the%20exodus%20project%20barnsley&epa=SEARCH_BOX

Recommended small businesses

https://skinkiss.org.uk/

https://favouritekafei.co.uk/?fbclid=IwAR1pW2
OJNWCtFdIpgU7WWp9JQiQDxbBxu4GfzBfr6648
snFYFERRYvGW7Ss

My Buy Me a Coffee website can be found here:

https://www.buymeacoffee.com/lynnedmnobl

The site contains a number of protocols as well
as current health related topics

ⁱ Cholesterol is a healing molecule and often levels which are deemed to be high is simply cholesterol responding to a need